MARBURG VIRUS DISEASE:
What you Need to Know about The Viral Disease

By

Robert M. Toller

Table of contents

Introduction

Marburg virus disease (MVD) is a rare but deadly disease caused by the Marburg virus. The disease was first identified in 1967 during an outbreak in Germany, and since then, several outbreaks have occurred in Africa. The virus is transmitted to humans through contact with infected animals or through human-to-human transmission.

MVD is a severe disease that causes symptoms such as fever, headache, muscle aches, vomiting, diarrhea, and bleeding from various parts of the body. The disease progresses rapidly, and patients can develop complications such as respiratory distress, shock, and organ failure. The fatality rate of MVD is high, with up to 88% of patients succumbing to the disease.

Due to the severity of the disease and the lack of effective treatment options, it is crucial to understand MVD and take steps to prevent its spread. This book aims to provide a comprehensive overview of Marburg virus disease, including its history, transmission, symptoms, diagnosis, prevention, and treatment.

In the following chapters, we will explore the nature of the Marburg virus, its history, and its impact on public health. We will also examine the symptoms of the disease and its diagnosis, as well as the measures that can be taken to prevent its spread. Furthermore, we will discuss the supportive care measures available to manage the disease and the experimental treatments currently being evaluated in clinical trials.

Overall, this book aims to provide a comprehensive guide to Marburg virus disease, including the latest research and recommendations for preventing and managing this deadly disease. It is our hope that this book will serve as a valuable resource for healthcare professionals, policymakers, researchers, and the general public alike, in their efforts to control the spread of this disease and protect public health.

Chapter 1: Introduction to Marburg Virus Disease

Marburg virus disease (MVD) is a highly infectious and deadly disease caused by the Marburg virus, a member of the Filoviridae family of viruses, which also includes the Ebola virus. The virus is named after the German city of Marburg, where the first known outbreak occurred in 1967. Since then, sporadic outbreaks of MVD have occurred in several African countries, including Angola, Democratic Republic of Congo, Kenya, South Africa, and Uganda.

The Marburg virus is believed to be endemic to fruit bats, which serve as a natural reservoir for the virus. The virus is transmitted to humans through contact with infected animals or animal products, such as bat droppings or fruit contaminated by bat urine or saliva. In some cases, the virus may also be transmitted from person to person through contact with infected blood, semen, or other bodily fluids.

MVD is a severe and often fatal disease, with a mortality rate of up to 90% in some outbreaks. The disease is characterized by fever, headache, muscle aches, and other flu-like symptoms, which may progress to severe hemorrhagic fever, causing bleeding from the eyes, nose, mouth, and other orifices. Other symptoms may include vomiting, diarrhea, and organ failure.

Although MVD is a rare disease, it poses a serious public health threat due to its high mortality rate, potential for rapid spread, and lack of effective treatments or vaccines. Outbreaks of MVD require a coordinated response from public health officials, health workers, and the affected communities to control the spread of the disease and provide care for the affected individuals. Ongoing research is needed to better understand the virus, develop effective treatments and vaccines, and prevent future outbreaks.

The first known outbreak of MVD occurred in 1967, when laboratory workers in Marburg, Germany, and Belgrade, Serbia, became ill after handling infected African green monkeys imported from Uganda for research purposes. The disease was named after the German city of Marburg where the first outbreak occurred. The virus responsible for the outbreak was later identified as a member of the Filoviridae family of viruses, which also includes the Ebola virus.

Since then, sporadic outbreaks of MVD have occurred in several African countries, mostly in remote areas where fruit bats, which are natural carriers of the virus, live. Outbreaks have been linked to activities such as visiting caves or mines where bats roost, handling sick or dead animals, or consuming contaminated fruits or other foods.

MVD is similar to Ebola virus disease in terms of its symptoms and mode of transmission. However, MVD is generally less contagious and has a lower case fatality rate than Ebola virus disease. Nonetheless, MVD is still a serious and potentially fatal disease, with a high mortality rate in some outbreaks. The disease can be difficult to diagnose and treat, and there is no specific treatment or vaccine currently available.

Outbreaks of MVD require a coordinated response from public health officials, health workers, and the affected communities to control the spread of the disease and provide care for the affected individuals. This involves implementing measures such as isolating infected individuals, tracing and monitoring contacts, implementing infection control measures in healthcare facilities, and providing supportive care for patients.

Preventing MVD requires reducing contact between humans and infected animals or animal products, such as bat droppings or fruit contaminated by bat urine or saliva. Health workers who care for MVD patients must take strict infection control measures, including wearing protective clothing, isolating patients, and disinfecting equipment and surfaces.

In summary, Marburg virus disease is a rare but serious disease caused by a highly infectious virus. While it is endemic to certain parts of Africa, the virus has the potential to spread to other regions of the world through travel and trade. Therefore, awareness of the signs and symptoms of MVD, prevention and control measures, and ongoing research efforts are crucial to prevent future outbreaks and manage the disease effectively.

Chapter 2: Signs and Symptoms of Marburg Virus Disease

Marburg virus disease (MVD) is a severe and often fatal disease caused by the Marburg virus. The symptoms of MVD can be similar to those of other viral illnesses, such as influenza or Ebola virus disease. However, MVD is characterized by a rapid onset of symptoms and a high mortality rate, with some outbreaks reporting a mortality rate of up to 90%.

The incubation period for MVD ranges from 2 to 21 days, with symptoms usually appearing between

5 to 10 days after exposure. The early symptoms of MVD are similar to those of the flu and may include:

Fever
Chills
Headache
Muscle aches
Weakness and fatigue
Nausea and vomiting
Diarrhea
Loss of appetite

As the disease progresses, more severe symptoms may develop, such as:

Severe hemorrhagic fever, causing bleeding from the eyes, nose, mouth, and other orifices

Jaundice (yellowing of the skin and eyes)

Rash

Chest pain

Difficulty breathing

Shock

Multi-organ failure

The severity of the symptoms can vary depending on the individual and the strain of the virus causing the outbreak. Some individuals may experience only mild symptoms, while others may develop severe hemorrhagic fever and die within a few days.

In addition to the physical symptoms, individuals affected by MVD may also experience psychological and emotional distress. Fear, anxiety, and confusion are common reactions to the disease, and can lead to social stigma and discrimination against survivors and their families.

It is important to note that the symptoms of MVD are similar to those of other viral illnesses, and a proper diagnosis can only be made through laboratory testing. Therefore, anyone who has been in contact with an infected individual or has traveled to an area where MVD has been reported and is experiencing symptoms should seek medical attention immediately.

In summary, the symptoms of MVD can range from mild flu-like symptoms to severe hemorrhagic fever, and can be fatal in some cases. Anyone experiencing symptoms should seek medical attention immediately, especially if they have traveled to areas where MVD has been reported or have had contact with infected individuals or animals.

It is important to note that the symptoms of MVD can overlap with those of other infectious diseases such as Ebola, Lassa fever, and Yellow fever. This can make it challenging to diagnose MVD early on, especially in regions where these diseases are endemic.

In some outbreaks, MVD has been known to cause severe hemorrhagic fever, which can lead to significant internal bleeding and shock. This is a life-threatening condition that requires immediate medical attention.

The risk of death from MVD is highest in individuals who develop severe hemorrhagic fever or multi-organ failure. Mortality rates have varied between different outbreaks, ranging from 24% to 88%. Survivors of MVD may experience long-term health problems, including hearing loss, vision problems, and joint pain.

It is important to note that the incubation period of MVD can vary from person to person, and symptoms may not appear until several days or even weeks after exposure to the virus. During this time, individuals can still transmit the virus to others through contact with bodily fluids.

Therefore, it is essential to take preventive measures to avoid exposure to the virus. These include avoiding contact with infected individuals, animals, or their bodily fluids, wearing protective clothing and equipment when caring for patients, and following strict infection control protocols.

Marburg virus disease is a severe and potentially fatal illness that can cause flu-like symptoms, hemorrhagic fever, and organ failure. Diagnosis can be challenging, as the symptoms can overlap with those of other infectious diseases. Prompt medical attention and strict infection control measures are essential to prevent the spread of the disease and provide appropriate care for affected individuals.

Chapter 3: Transmission and Prevention of Marburg Virus Disease

Marburg virus disease (MVD) is caused by the Marburg virus, which is a member of the filovirus family, along with Ebola virus. The virus is primarily transmitted through contact with the bodily fluids of infected individuals or animals, such as blood, urine, feces, vomit, and semen.

Transmission of the virus can occur through:

Direct contact with infected bodily fluids, such as through broken skin or mucous membranes

Contact with contaminated objects or surfaces, such as medical equipment, needles, or bedding

Contact with infected animals, such as monkeys or bats, through hunting or consumption of their meat

Person-to-person transmission through close contact with infected individuals, such as caring for sick family members or healthcare workers providing medical care.

The risk of transmission is highest during the late stages of the disease, when the virus is present in high concentrations in bodily fluids.

However, the virus can also be present in bodily fluids during the early stages of the disease, which can make it challenging to control its spread.

Prevention measures are essential to control the spread of MVD. These include:

Avoiding contact with infected individuals, animals, or their bodily fluids

Wearing protective clothing and equipment, such as gloves, masks, and goggles, when caring for infected individuals or handling infected materials

Following strict infection control protocols, such as washing hands frequently with soap and water, using disinfectants to clean surfaces, and disposing of contaminated materials safely

Isolating infected individuals to prevent person-to-person transmission

Screening travelers for symptoms of the disease and restricting travel from affected areas.

There is currently no specific treatment or vaccine for MVD, and management of the disease is mainly supportive, focusing on alleviating symptoms and preventing complications. Supportive care may include intravenous fluids, electrolyte replacement, oxygen therapy, and treatment for secondary infections.

Research is ongoing to develop treatments and vaccines for MVD. Several experimental treatments, such as monoclonal antibodies and antiviral drugs, have shown promise in animal studies and are being tested in clinical trials.

In summary, Marburg virus disease is primarily transmitted through contact with the bodily fluids of infected individuals or animals. Prevention measures, such as avoiding contact with infected individuals or their bodily fluids, wearing protective equipment, and following strict infection control protocols, are essential to control the spread of the disease. There is currently no specific treatment or vaccine for MVD, and management of the disease is mainly supportive.

In addition to the prevention measures mentioned in the previous section, there are several other strategies that can be used to control outbreaks of MVD.

Contact tracing is an essential component of outbreak control. This involves identifying and monitoring individuals who have had contact with infected individuals to detect new cases early on and prevent further spread of the disease.

Community engagement and education are also critical to controlling the spread of MVD. This includes raising awareness about the signs and symptoms of the disease, promoting good hygiene practices, and addressing cultural and traditional practices that may increase the risk of transmission.

Surveillance and early detection systems are also essential to detecting and responding to outbreaks quickly. This involves establishing mechanisms for detecting and reporting suspected cases of the disease, testing samples for the virus, and implementing control measures as soon as possible.

International cooperation and collaboration are also essential to controlling outbreaks of MVD. This includes sharing information and resources, providing technical assistance to affected countries, and supporting research efforts to develop treatments and vaccines for the disease.

The World Health Organization (WHO) plays a critical role in coordinating global efforts to control outbreaks of MVD. The organization provides technical guidance and support to affected countries, facilitates the exchange of information and resources, and mobilizes international resources to respond to outbreaks quickly.

In conclusion, controlling outbreaks of Marburg virus disease requires a multifaceted approach that involves prevention measures, early detection and surveillance, community engagement and education, and international cooperation and collaboration. These efforts are essential to controlling the spread of the disease, preventing complications, and reducing the risk of death.

Chapter 4: Prevention of Marburg Virus Disease

Marburg virus disease (MVD) is a severe illness caused by the Marburg virus, and there is currently no specific treatment or vaccine available for the disease. As a result, prevention is critical to controlling the spread of the disease and reducing the risk of illness and death.

The following are some of the most effective prevention measures that can be taken to reduce the risk of contracting MVD:

Avoid contact with infected individuals or animals: Marburg virus is primarily transmitted through contact with the bodily fluids of infected individuals or animals, including blood, urine, feces, vomit, and semen. Therefore, it is essential to avoid contact with infected individuals or animals to prevent the spread of the disease.

Wear protective clothing and equipment: If contact with infected individuals or materials is unavoidable, it is essential to wear appropriate protective clothing and equipment, such as gloves, masks, and goggles, to reduce the risk of infection.

Practice good hygiene: Frequent hand washing with soap and water, particularly after handling materials that may be contaminated with the virus, is an essential step in preventing the spread of MVD.

Follow infection control procedures: Individuals who come into contact with infected individuals or materials must follow strict infection control procedures to prevent the spread of the disease. This may include using disinfectants to clean surfaces, isolating infected individuals, and properly disposing of contaminated materials.

Avoid consumption of bushmeat: Marburg virus can be transmitted to humans through the consumption of infected bushmeat, including monkey and bat meat. Therefore, avoiding the consumption of bushmeat is an essential step in preventing the spread of the disease.

Screen and isolate travelers: Screening individuals for symptoms of MVD and restricting travel from affected areas can help prevent the spread of the disease to new locations.

Promote community awareness: Raising awareness about the signs and symptoms of MVD, promoting good hygiene practices, and addressing cultural and traditional practices that may increase the risk of transmission can help prevent the spread of the disease in communities.

In conclusion, prevention is the most effective way to control the spread of Marburg virus disease. Avoiding contact with infected individuals or animals, wearing protective clothing and equipment, practicing good hygiene, following infection control procedures, avoiding consumption of bushmeat, screening and isolating travelers, and promoting community awareness are all essential measures that can be taken to prevent the spread of the disease.

In addition to the prevention measures listed in the previous section, there are other strategies that can be employed to reduce the risk of contracting Marburg virus disease.

One such strategy is the development of a vaccine. Currently, there is no licensed vaccine for MVD, but research is ongoing to develop one. Several candidate vaccines have shown promise in animal studies and are being evaluated in clinical trials.

Another strategy is the development of antiviral drugs to treat MVD. Several experimental drugs have shown promise in laboratory studies, and clinical trials are ongoing to evaluate their safety and efficacy in humans.

Effective outbreak control measures are also essential in preventing the spread of MVD. This includes the rapid identification and isolation of infected individuals, contact tracing, and the implementation of strict infection control measures in healthcare settings.

Surveillance systems for detecting and reporting suspected cases of MVD, along with laboratory capacity for testing samples for the virus, are also critical to preventing the spread of the disease.

International collaboration is also crucial in preventing the spread of MVD. The World Health Organization (WHO) coordinates global efforts to control outbreaks of the disease, provides technical guidance and support to affected countries, and mobilizes international resources to respond to outbreaks quickly.

In conclusion, while there is no specific treatment or vaccine available for Marburg virus disease, prevention measures such as avoiding contact with infected individuals or animals, wearing protective clothing and equipment, practicing good hygiene, and promoting community awareness can significantly reduce the risk of contracting the disease. Additionally, the development of a vaccine and antiviral drugs, effective outbreak control measures, surveillance systems, and international collaboration are essential in preventing the spread of the disease.

Chapter 5: Treatment of Marburg Virus Disease

Currently, there is no specific treatment available for MVD, and management of the disease is primarily supportive.

Supportive care measures include:

Fluid and electrolyte management: Patients with MVD often experience vomiting and diarrhea, which can lead to dehydration and electrolyte imbalances. Therefore, providing fluids and electrolytes is critical to maintaining the patient's hydration and electrolyte balance.

Treatment of complications: Patients with MVD may develop complications, such as respiratory distress, hypotension, and shock. These complications must be promptly recognized and treated to improve the patient's chances of survival.

Pain management: Patients with MVD may experience severe pain, and appropriate pain management is essential to alleviate their discomfort.

Nutritional support: Patients with MVD may experience loss of appetite and weight loss. Therefore, providing adequate nutrition is critical to maintain the patient's nutritional status and support their recovery.

Infection prevention and control: Strict infection prevention and control measures are essential to prevent the spread of the virus to healthcare workers and other patients.

Experimental treatments for MVD are currently being evaluated in clinical trials. These treatments include the use of monoclonal antibodies, antiviral drugs, and convalescent plasma, which is obtained from patients who have recovered from the disease and contains antibodies against the virus.

The use of these treatments is still experimental, and their safety and efficacy in humans are not yet fully understood. Therefore, they should only be used under strict clinical trial conditions.

There is no specific treatment available for Marburg virus disease, and management of the disease is primarily supportive. Fluid and electrolyte management, treatment of complications, pain management, nutritional support, and infection prevention and control are critical to supporting the patient's recovery. Experimental treatments for MVD are currently being evaluated in clinical trials, but their safety and efficacy in humans are not yet fully understood.

Conclusion:

Marburg virus disease (MVD) is a rare but deadly disease that poses a significant public health threat. Although the disease has been identified for over five decades, there is still much that is not understood about it, and there are currently no licensed vaccines or specific treatments available.

This book has provided a comprehensive overview of MVD, including its history, transmission, symptoms, diagnosis, prevention, and treatment. We have explored the nature of the Marburg virus and its impact on public health, as well as the measures that can be taken to prevent its spread.

While there are currently no specific treatments for MVD, supportive care measures are available to manage the disease's symptoms. Moreover, ongoing research into experimental treatments such as monoclonal antibodies, antiviral drugs, and convalescent plasma is showing promising results.

International collaboration is also critical in preventing the spread of the disease, and the World Health

Organization (WHO) plays a vital role in coordinating global efforts to control outbreaks of MVD.

In conclusion, this book provides a valuable resource for healthcare professionals, policymakers, researchers, and the general public in their efforts to understand and control the spread of Marburg virus disease. We hope that this book will increase awareness of MVD and encourage the development of effective treatments and vaccines to protect against future outbreaks. With continued research, collaboration, and implementation of prevention measures, we can reduce the impact of MVD on public health.